THE KET RESET D...

How burn fat forever

Melissa Cameron

Sommario

INTRODUCTION

Do you want to make a change in your life? Do you want to become a healthier person who can enjoy a new and improved life? Then, you are definitely in the right place. You are about to discover a wonderful and very healthy diet that has changed millions of lives. We are talking about the Ketogenic diet, a lifestyle that will mesmerize you and that will make you a new person in no time.

So, let's sit back, relax and find out more about the Ketogenic diet.

A keto diet is a low carb one. This is the first and one of the most important things you should now. During such a diet, your body makes ketones in your liver and these are used as energy.

Your body will produce less insulin and glucose and a state of ketosis is induced.

Ketosis is a natural process that appears when our food intake is lower than usual. The body will soon adapt to this state and therefore you will be able to lose weight in no time but you will also become healthier and your physical and mental performances will improve.

Your blood sugar levels will improve and you won't be predisposed to diabetes. Also, epilepsy and heart diseases can be prevented if you are on a Ketogenic diet. Your cholesterol will improve and you will feel amazing in no time.

How does that sound?

A Ketogenic diet is simple and easy to follow as long as you follow some simple rules. You don't need to make huge changes but there are some things you should know.

So, here goes!

BREAKFAST

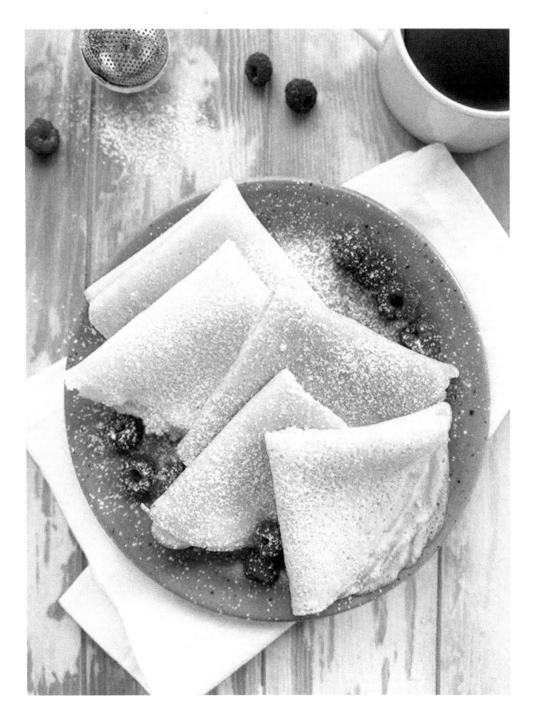

Amazing Breakfast In A Glass

Don't bother making something complex for breakfast! Try this amazing keto drink!

Preparation time: 3 minutes **Cooking time:** 0 minutes **Servings:** 2

Ingredients:

10 ounces canned coconut milk

1 cup favorite greens

¼ cup cocoa nibs

1 cup water

1 cup cherries, frozen

¼ cup cocoa powder

1 small avocado, pitted and peeled

¼ teaspoon turmeric

Directions:

1. In your blender, mix coconut milk with avocado, cocoa powder, cherries and turmeric and blend well.

2. Add water, greens and cocoa nibs, blend for 2 minutes more, pour into glasses and serve.

Enjoy!

Nutrition: calories 100, fat 3, fiber 2, carbs 3, protein 5

Delicious Chicken Quiche

It's so delicious that you will ask for more!

Preparation time: 10 minutes **Cooking time:** 45 minutes **Servings:** 5

Ingredients:

7 eggs

2 cups almond flour

2 tablespoons coconut oil

Salt and black pepper to the taste

2 zucchinis, grated

½ cup heavy cream

1 teaspoon fennel seeds

1 teaspoon oregano, dried

1 pound chicken meat, ground

Directions:

1. In your food processor, blend almond flour with a pinch of salt.

2. Add 1 egg and coconut oil and blend well.

3. Place dough in a greased pie pan and press well on the bottom.

4. Heat up a pan over medium heat, add chicken meat, brown for a couple of minutes, take off heat and leave aside.

5. In a bowl, mix 6 eggs with salt, pepper, oregano, cream and fennel seeds and whisk well.

6. Add chicken meat and stir again.

7. Pour this into pie crust, spread, introduce in the oven at 350 degrees F and bake for 40 minutes.

8. Leave the pie to cool down a bit before slicing and serving it for breakfast!

Enjoy!

Nutrition: calories 300, fat 23, fiber 3, carbs 4, protein 18

Delicious Steak And Eggs

This is so rich and hearty! Dare and try this for breakfast tomorrow!

Preparation time: 10 minutes **Cooking time:** 10 minutes **Servings:** 1

Ingredients:

4 ounces sirloin

1 small avocado, pitted, peeled and sliced

3 eggs

1 tablespoon ghee

Salt and black pepper to the taste

Directions:

1. Heat up a pan with the ghee over medium high heat, crack eggs into the pan and cook them as you wish.

2. Season with salt and pepper, take off heat and transfer to a plate.

3. Heat up another pan over medium high heat, add sirloin, cook for 4 minutes, take off heat, leave aside to cool down and cut into thin strips.

4. Season with salt and pepper to the taste and place next to the eggs.

5. Add avocado slices on the side and serve.

Enjoy!

Nutrition: calories 500, fat 34, fiber 10, carbs 3, protein 40

Amazing Chicken Omelet

It tastes amazing and it looks incredible! It's perfect!

Preparation time: 10 minutes **Cooking time:** 10 minutes **Servings:** 1

Ingredients:

1 ounce rotisserie chicken, shredded

1 teaspoon mustard

1 tablespoon homemade mayonnaise

1 tomato, chopped

2 bacon slices, cooked and crumbled

2 eggs

1 small avocado, pitted, peeled and chopped

Salt and black pepper to the taste

Directions:

1. In a bowl, mix eggs with some salt and pepper and whisk gently.

2. Heat up a pan over medium heat, spray with some cooking oil, add eggs and cook your omelet for 5 minutes.

3. Add chicken, avocado, tomato, bacon, mayo and mustard on one half of the omelet.

4. Fold omelet, cover pan and cook for 5 minutes more.

5. Transfer to a plate and serve.

Enjoy!

Nutrition: calories 400, fat 32, fiber 6, carbs 4, protein 25

Simple Smoothie Bowl

It's one of the best keto breakfast ideas ever!

Preparation time: 5 minutes **Cooking time:** 0 minutes **Servings:** 1

Ingredients:

2 ice cubes

1 tablespoon coconut oil

2 tablespoons heavy cream

1 cup spinach

½ cup almond milk

1 teaspoon protein powder

4 raspberries

1 tablespoon coconut ,shredded

4 walnuts

1 teaspoon chia seeds

Directions:

1. In your blender, mix milk with spinach, cream, ice, protein powder and coconut oil, blend well and transfer to a bowl.

2. Top your bowl with raspberries, coconut, walnuts and chia seeds and serve.

Enjoy!

Nutrition: calories 450, fat 34, fiber 4, carbs 4, protein 35

Feta Omelet

The combination of ingredients is just wonderful!

Preparation time: 10 minutes **Cooking time:** 10 minutes **Servings:** 1

Ingredients:

3 eggs

1 tablespoon ghee

1 ounce feta cheese, crumbled

1 tablespoon heavy cream

1 tablespoon jarred pesto

Salt and black pepper to the taste

Directions:

1. In a bowl, mix eggs with heavy cream, salt and pepper and whisk well.

2. Heat up a pan with the ghee over medium high heat, add whisked eggs, spread into the pan and cook your omelet until it's fluffy.

3. Sprinkle cheese and spread pesto on your omelet, fold in half, cover pan and cook for 5 minutes more.

4. Transfer omelet to a plate and serve.

Enjoy!

Nutrition: calories 500, fat 43, fiber 6, carbs 3, protein 30

Breakfast Meatloaf

This is something worth trying as soon as possible!

Preparation time: 10 minutes **Cooking time:** 35 minutes **Servings:** 4

Ingredients:

1 teaspoon ghee

1 small yellow onion, chopped

1 pound sweet sausage, chopped

6 eggs

1 cup cheddar cheese, shredded

4 ounces cream cheese, soft

Salt and black pepper to the taste

2 tablespoons scallions, chopped

Directions:

1. In a bowl, mix eggs with salt, pepper, onion, sausage and half of the cream and whisk well.

2. Grease a meatloaf with the ghee, pour sausage and eggs mix, introduce in the oven at 350 degrees F and bake for 30 minutes.

3. Take meatloaf out of the oven, leave aside for a couple of minutes, spread the rest of the cream cheese on top and sprinkle scallions and cheddar cheese all over.

4. Introduce meatloaf in the oven again and bake for 5 minutes more.

5. After the time has passed, broil meatloaf for 3 minutes, leave it aside to cool down a bit, slice and serve it.

Enjoy!

Nutrition: calories 560, fat 32, fiber 1, carbs 6, protein 45

Breakfast Tuna Salad

You will love this Ketogenic breakfast from now on!

Preparation time: 10 minutes **Cooking time:** 0 minutes **Servings:** 4

Ingredients:

2 tablespoons sour cream

12 ounces tuna in olive oil

4 leeks, finely chopped

Salt and black pepper to the taste

A pinch of chili flakes

1 tablespoon capers

8 tablespoons homemade mayonnaise

Directions:

1. In a salad bowl, mix tuna with capers, salt, pepper, leeks, chili flakes, sour cream and mayo.

2. Stir well and serve with some crispy bread.

Enjoy!

Nutrition: calories 160, fat 2, fiber 1, carbs 2, protein 6

Incredible Breakfast Salad In A Jar

You can even take this at the office!

Preparation time: 10 minutes **Cooking time:** 0 minutes **Servings:** 1

Ingredients:

1 ounce favorite greens

1 ounce red bell pepper, chopped

1 ounce cherry tomatoes, halved

4 ounces rotisserie chicken, roughly chopped

4 tablespoons extra virgin olive oil

½ scallion, chopped

1 ounce cucumber, chopped

Salt and black pepper to the taste

Directions:

1. In a bowl, mix greens with bell pepper, tomatoes, scallion, cucumber, salt, pepper and olive oil and toss to coat well.

2. Transfer this to a jar, top with chicken pieces and serve for breakfast.

Enjoy!

Nutrition: calories 180, fat 12, fiber 4, carbs 5, protein 17

Delicious Naan Bread And Butter

Try this special keto breakfast! It's so easy to make!

Preparation time: 10 minutes **Cooking time:** 10 minutes **Servings:** 6

Ingredients:

7 tablespoons coconut oil

¾ cup coconut flour

2 tablespoons psyllium powder

½ teaspoon baking powder

Salt to the taste

2 cups hot water

Some coconut oil for frying

2 garlic cloves, minced

3.5 ounces ghee

Directions:

1. In a bowl, mix coconut flour with baking powder, salt and psyllium powder and stir.

2. Add 7 tablespoons coconut oil and the hot water and start kneading your dough.

3. Leave aside for 5 minutes, divide into 6 balls and flatten them on a working surface.

4. Heat up a pan with some coconut oil over medium high heat, add naan breads to the pan, fry them until they are golden and transfer them to a plate.

5. Heat up a pan with the ghee over medium high heat, add garlic, salt and pepper, stir and cook for 2 minutes.

6. Brush naan breads with this mix and pour the rest into a bowl.

7. Serve in the morning.

Enjoy!

Nutrition: calories 140, fat 9, fiber 2, carbs 3, protein 4

SIDE DISH

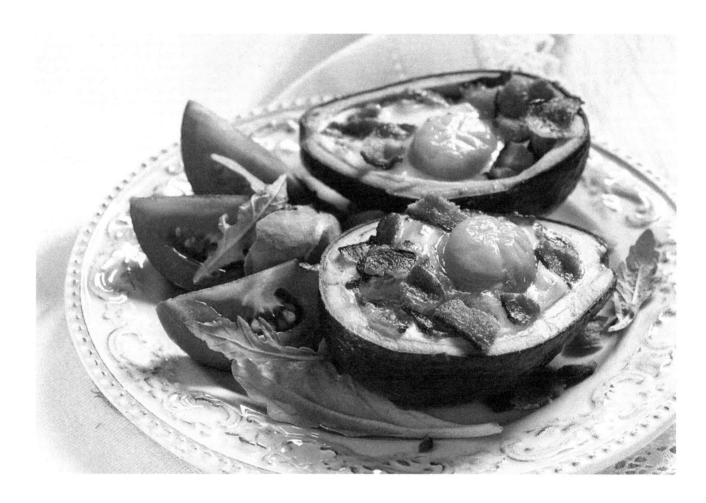

Asian Side Salad

It has a delicious and amazing flavor! It goes perfectly with some keto shrimp!

Preparation time: 30 minutes **Cooking time:** 10 minutes **Servings:** 4

Ingredients:

1 big cucumber, thinly sliced

1 spring onion, chopped

2 tablespoons coconut oil

1 packet Asian noodles

1 tablespoon balsamic vinegar

1 tablespoon sesame oil

¼ teaspoon red pepper flakes

Salt and black pepper to the taste

1 teaspoon sesame seeds

Directions:

1. Cook noodles according to package instructions, drain and rinse them

well.

2. Heat up a pan with the coconut oil over medium high heat, add noodles, cover pan and fry them for 5 minutes until they are crispy enough.

3. Transfer them to paper towels and drain grease.

4. In a bowl, mix cucumber slices with spring onion, pepper flakes, vinegar, sesame oil, sesame seeds, salt, pepper and noodles.

5. Toss to coat well, keep in the fridge for 30 minutes and serve as a side for some grilled shrimp.

Enjoy!

Nutrition: calories 400, fat 34, fiber 2, carbs 4, protein 2

Mixed Veggie Dish

Serve with a tasty keto steak!

Preparation time: 10 minutes **Cooking time:** 10 minutes **Servings:** 4

Ingredients:

14 ounces mushrooms, sliced

3 ounces broccoli florets

3.5 ounces sugar snap peas

6 tablespoons olive oil

Salt and black pepper to the taste

3 ounces bell pepper, cut into strips

3 ounces spinach, torn

2 tablespoons garlic, minced

2 tablespoons pumpkin seeds

A pinch of red pepper flakes

Directions:

1. Heat up a pan with the oil over medium high heat, add garlic, stir and cook for 1 minute.

2. Add mushrooms, stir and cook for 3 minutes more.

3. Add broccoli and stir everything.

4. Add snap peas and peppers and stir again.

5. Add salt, pepper, pumpkin seeds and pepper flakes, stir and cook for a few minutes.

6. Add spinach, stir gently, cook for a couple of minutes, divide between plates and serve as a side dish.

Enjoy!

Nutrition: calories 247, fat 23, fiber 4, carbs 3, protein 7

Amazing Cauliflower Polenta

This should be very interesting! Let's learn how to prepare it!

Preparation time: 10 minutes **Cooking time:** 1 hour **Servings:** 2

Ingredients:

1 cauliflower head, florets separated and chopped

¼ cup hazelnuts

1 tablespoon olive oil + 2 teaspoons extra virgin olive oil

1 small yellow onion, chopped

3 cups shiitake mushrooms, chopped

4 garlic cloves

3 tablespoons nutritional yeast

½ cup water

Chopped parsley for serving

Directions:

1. Spread hazelnuts on a lined baking sheet, introduce in the oven at 350 degrees F and bake for 10 minutes.

2. Take hazelnuts out of the oven, leave them to cool down, chop and leave aside for now.

3. Spread cauliflower florets on the baking sheet, drizzle 1 teaspoon oil, introduce in the oven at 400 degrees F and bake for 30 minutes.

4. In a bowl, mix oil with ½ teaspoon oil and toss to coat.

5. Put garlic cloves on a tin foil, drizzle ½ teaspoon oil and wrap.

6. Spread onion next to cauliflower, also add wrapped garlic to the baking sheet, introduce in the oven everything and bake for 20 minutes.

7. Heat up a pan with the rest of the oil over medium high heat,

add mushrooms, stir and cook for 8 minutes.

8. Take cauliflower out of the oven and transfer to your food processor.

9. Unwrap garlic, peel and also add to the food processor.

10. Add onion, yeast, salt and pepper and blend everything well.

11. Divide polenta on plates, top with mushrooms, hazelnuts and parsley and serve as a side.

Enjoy!

Nutrition: calories 342, fat 21, fiber 12, carbs 3, protein 14

Amazing Side Dish

This will totally surprise you!

Preparation time: 10 minutes **Cooking time:** 4 hours and 20 minutes

Servings:

8

Ingredients:

2 cups almond flour

2 tablespoons whey protein powder

¼ cup coconut flour

½ teaspoon garlic powder

2 teaspoons baking powder

1 and ¼ cups cheddar cheese, shredded

2 eggs

¼ cup melted ghee

¾ cup water

For the stuffing:

½ cup yellow onion, chopped

2 tablespoons ghee

1 red bell pepper, chopped

1 jalapeno pepper, chopped

Salt and black pepper to the taste

12 ounces sausage, chopped

2 eggs

¾ cup chicken stock

¼ cup whipping cream

Directions:

1. In a bowl, mix coconut flour with whey protein, almond flour, garlic powder, baking powder and 1 cup cheddar cheese and

stir everything.

2. Add water, 2 eggs and ¼ cup ghee and stir well.

3. Transfer this to a greased baking pan, sprinkle the rest of the cheddar cheese, introduce in the oven at 325 degrees F and bake for 30 minutes.

4. Leave the bread to cool down for 15 minutes and cube it.

5. Spread bread cubes on a lined baking sheet, introduce in the oven at 200 degrees F and bake for 3 hours.

6. Take bread cubes out of the oven and leave aside for now.

7. Heat up a pan with 2 tablespoons ghee over medium heat, add onion, stir and cook for 4 minutes.

8. Add jalapeno and red bell pepper, stir and cook for 5 minutes.

9. Add salt and pepper, stir and transfer everything to a bowl.

10. Heat up the same pan over medium heat, add sausage, stir and cook for 10 minutes.

11. Transfer to the bowl with the veggies, also add stock, bread and stir everything.

12. In a separate bowl, whisk 2 eggs with some salt, pepper and whipping cream.

13. Add this to sausage and bread mix, stir, transfer to a greased baking pan, introduce in the oven at 325 degrees F and bake for 30 minutes.

14. Serve hot as a side.

Enjoy!

Nutrition: calories 340, fat 4, fiber 6, carbs 3.4, protein 7

Special Mushrooms

It's so yummy! You have to try it to see!

Preparation time: 10 minutes **Cooking time:** 30 minutes **Servings:** 4

Ingredients:

4 tablespoons ghee

16 ounces baby mushrooms

Salt and black pepper to the taste

3 tablespoons onion, dried

3 tablespoons parsley flakes

1 teaspoon garlic powder

Directions:

1. In a bowl, mix parsley flakes with onion, salt, pepper and garlic powder and stir.

2. In another bowl, mix mushroom with melted ghee and toss to coat.

3. Add seasoning mix, toss well, spread on a lined baking sheet, introduce in the oven at 300 degrees F and bake for 30 minutes.

4. Serve as a side dish for a tasty keto roast.

Enjoy!

Nutrition: calories 152, fat 12, fiber 5, carbs 6, protein 4

Green Beans And Tasty Vinaigrette

You will find this keto side dish really amazing!

Preparation time: 10 minutes **Cooking time:** 12 minutes **Serving:** 8

Ingredients:

2 ounces chorizo, chopped

1 garlic clove, minced

1 teaspoon lemon juice

2 teaspoons smoked paprika

½ cup coconut vinegar

4 tablespoons macadamia nut oil

¼ teaspoon coriander, ground

Salt and black pepper to the taste

2 tablespoons coconut oil

2 tablespoons beef stock

2 pound green beans

Directions:

1. In a blender, mix chorizo with salt, pepper, vinegar, garlic, lemon juice, paprika and coriander and pulse well.

2. Add the stock and the macadamia nut oil and blend again.

3. Heat up a pan with the coconut oil over medium heat, add green beans and chorizo mix, stir and cook for 10 minutes.

4. Divide between plates and serve.

Enjoy!

Nutrition: calories 160, fat 12, fiber 4, carbs 6, protein 4

Braised Eggplant Side Dish

Try this Vietnamese keto side dish!

Preparation time: 10 minutes **Cooking time:** 15 minutes **Servings:** 4
Ingredients:

1 big Asian eggplant, cut into medium pieces

1 yellow onion, thinly sliced

2 tablespoon vegetable oil

2 teaspoons garlic, minced

½ cup Vietnamese sauce

½ cup water

2 teaspoons chili paste

¼ cup coconut milk

4 green onions, chopped

For the Vietnamese sauce:

1 teaspoon palm sugar

½ cup chicken stock

2 tablespoons fish sauce

Directions:

1. Put stock in a pan and heat up over medium heat.

2. Add sugar and fish sauce, stir well and leave aside for now.

3. Heat up a pan over medium high heat, add eggplant pieces, brown them for 2 minutes and transfer to a plate.

4. Heat up the pan again with the oil over medium high heat, add yellow onion and garlic, stir and cook for 2 minutes.

5. Return eggplant pieces and cook for 2 minutes.

6. Add water, the Vietnamese sauce you've made earlier, chili paste and coconut milk, stir and cook for 5 minutes.

7. Add green onions, stir, cook for 1 minute more, transfer to

plates and serve as a side dish.

Enjoy!

Nutrition: calories 142, fat 7, fiber 4, carbs 5, protein 3

Cheddar Soufflés

If you are on a Ketogenic diet, then you must really try this side dish! Serve with a steak on the side!

Preparation time: 10 minutes **Cooking time:** 25 minutes **Servings:** 8

Ingredients:¾ cup heavy cream

2 cups cheddar cheese, shredded

6 eggs

Salt and black pepper to the taste

¼ teaspoon cream of tartar

A pinch of cayenne pepper

½ teaspoon xanthan gum

1 teaspoon mustard powder

¼ cup chives, chopped

½ cup almond flour

Cooking spray

Directions:

1. In a bowl, mix almond flour with salt, pepper, mustard, xanthan gum and cayenne and whisk well.

2. Add cheese, cream, chives, eggs and cream of tartar and whisk well again.

3. Grease 8 ramekins with cooking spray, pour cheddar and chives mix, introduce in the oven at 350 degrees F and bake for 25 minutes.

4. Serve your soufflés with a tasty keto steak.

Enjoy!

Nutrition: calories 288, fat 23, fiber 1, carbs 3.3, protein 14

Tasty Cauliflower Side Salad

This is much better than you could ever imagine!

Preparation time: 10 minutes **Cooking time:** 5 minutes **Servings:** 10

Ingredients:

21 ounces cauliflower, florets separated

Salt and black pepper to the taste

1 cup red onion, chopped

1 cup celery, chopped

2 tablespoons cider vinegar

1 teaspoon splenda

4 eggs, hard-boiled, peeled and chopped

1 cup mayonnaise

1 tablespoon water

Directions:

1. Put cauliflower florets in a heatproof bowl, add the water, cover and cook in your microwave for 5 minutes.

2. Leave aside for another 5 minutes and transfer to a salad bowl.

3. Add celery, eggs and onions and stir gently.

4. In a bowl, mix mayo with salt, pepper, splenda and vinegar and whisk well.

5. Add this to salad, toss to coat well and serve right away with a side salad.

Enjoy!

Nutrition: calories 211, fat 20, fiber 2, carbs 3, protein 4

Amazing Rice

Don't worry! It's not made with actual rice!

Preparation time: 10 minutes **Cooking time:** 30 minutes **Servings:** 4

Ingredients:

1 cauliflower head, florets separated

Salt and black pepper to the taste

10 ounces coconut milk

½ cup water

2 ginger slices

2 tablespoons coconut shreds, toasted

Directions:

1. Put cauliflower in your food processor and blend.

2. Transfer cauliflower rice to a kitchen towel, press well and leave aside.

3. Heat up a pot with the coconut milk over medium heat.

4. Add the water and ginger, stir and bring to a simmer.

5. Add cauliflower, stir and cook for 30 minutes.

6. Discard ginger, add salt, pepper and coconut shreds, stir gently, divide between plates and serve as a side for a poultry based dish.

Enjoy!

Nutrition: calories 108, fat 3, fiber 6, carbs 5, protein 9

APPETIZERS

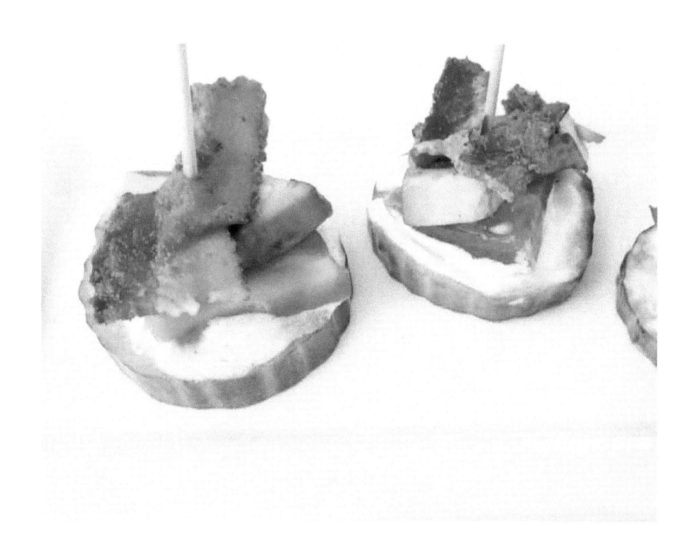

Delicious Cucumber Cups

Get ready to taste something really elegant and delicious!

Preparation time: 10 minutes **Cooking time:** 0 minutes **Servings:** 24

Ingredients:

2 cucumbers, peeled, cut into ¾ inch slices and some of the seeds scooped out

½ cup sour cream

Salt and white pepper to the taste

6 ounces smoked salmon, flaked

1/3 cup cilantro, chopped

2 teaspoons lime juice

1 tablespoon lime zest

A pinch of cayenne pepper

Directions:

1. In a bowl mix salmon with salt, pepper, cayenne, sour cream, lime juice and zest and cilantro and stir well.

2. Fill each cucumber cup with this salmon mix, arrange on a platter and serve as a keto appetizer.

Enjoy!

Nutrition: calories 30, fat 11, fiber 1, carbs 1, protein 2

Caviar Salad

This is so elegant! It's so delicious and sophisticated!

Preparation time: 6 minutes **Cooking time:** 0 minutes **Servings:** 16

Ingredients:

8 eggs, hard-boiled, peeled and mashed with a fork

4 ounces black caviar

4 ounces red caviar

Salt and black pepper to the taste

1 yellow onion, finely chopped

¾ cup mayonnaise

Some toast baguette slices for serving

Directions:

1. In a bowl, mix mashed eggs with mayo, salt, pepper and onion and stir well.

2. Spread eggs salad on toasted baguette slices, and top each with caviar.

Enjoy!

Nutrition: calories 122, fat 8, fiber 1, carbs 4, protein 7

Marinated Kebabs

This is the perfect appetizer for a summer barbecue!

Preparation time: 20 minutes **Cooking time:** 10 minutes **Servings:** 6

Ingredients:

1 red bell pepper, cut into chunks

1 green bell pepper, cut into chunks

1 orange bell pepper, cut into chunks

2 pounds sirloin steak, cut into medium cubes

4 garlic cloves, minced

1 red onion, cut into chunks

Salt and black pepper to the taste

2 tablespoons Dijon mustard

2 and ½ tablespoons Worcestershire sauce

¼ cup tamari sauce

¼ cup lemon juice

½ cup olive oil

Directions:

1. In a bowl, mix Worcestershire sauce with salt, pepper, garlic, mustard, tamari, lemon juice and oil and whisk very well.

2. Add beef, bell peppers and onion chunks to this mix, toss to coat and leave aside for a few minutes.

3. Arrange bell pepper, meat cubes and onion chunks on skewers alternating colors, place them on your preheated grill over medium high heat, cook for 5 minutes on each side, transfer to a platter and serve as a summer keto appetizer.

Enjoy!

Nutrition: calories 246, fat 12, fiber 1, carbs 4, protein 26

Simple Zucchini Rolls

You've got to try this simple and very tasty appetizer as soon as possible!

Preparation time: 10 minutes **Cooking time:** 5 minutes **Servings:** 24

Ingredients:

2 tablespoons olive oil

3 zucchinis, thinly sliced

24 basil leaves

2 tablespoons mint, chopped

1 and 1/3 cup ricotta cheese

Salt and black pepper to the taste

¼ cup basil, chopped

Tomato sauce for serving

Directions:

1. Brush zucchini slices with the olive oil, season with salt and pepper on both sides, place them on preheated grill over medium heat, cook them for 2 minutes, flip and cook for another 2 minutes.

2. Place zucchini slices on a plate and leave aside for now.

3. In a bowl, mix ricotta with chopped basil, mint, salt and pepper and stir well.

4. Spread this over zucchini slices, divide whole basil leaves as well, roll and serve as an appetizer with some tomato sauce on the side.

Enjoy!

Nutrition: calories 40, fat 3, fiber 0.3, carbs 1, protein 2

Simple Green Crackers

These are real fun to make and they taste amazing!

Preparation time: 10 minutes **Cooking time:** 24 hours **Servings:** 6

Ingredients:

2 cups flax seed, ground

2 cups flax seed, soaked overnight and drained

4 bunches kale, chopped

1 bunch basil, chopped

½ bunch celery, chopped

4 garlic cloves, minced

1/3 cup olive oil

Directions:

1. In your food processor mix ground flaxseed with celery, kale, basil and garlic and blend well.

2. Add oil and soaked flaxseed and blend again.

3. Spread this on a tray, cut into medium crackers, introduce in your dehydrator and dry for 24 hours at 115 degrees F, turning them halfway.

4. Arrange them on a platter and serve.

Enjoy!

Nutrition: calories 100, fat 1, fiber 2, carbs 1, protein 4

Cheese And Pesto Terrine

This looks so amazing and it tastes great!

Preparation time: 30 minutes **Cooking time:** 0 minutes **Servings:** 10

Ingredients:½ cup heavy cream

10 ounces goat cheese, crumbled

3 tablespoons basil pesto

Salt and black pepper to the taste

5 sun-dried tomatoes, chopped

¼ cup pine nuts, toasted and chopped

1 tablespoons pine nuts, toasted and chopped

Directions:

1. In a bowl, mix goat cheese with the heavy cream, salt and pepper and stir using your mixer.

2. Spoon half of this mix into a lined bowl and spread.

3. Add pesto on top and also spread.

4. Add another layer of cheese, then add sun dried tomatoes and ¼ cup pine nuts.

5. Spread one last layer of cheese and top with 1 tablespoon pine nuts.

6. Keep in the fridge for a while, turn upside down on a plate and serve.

Enjoy!

Nutrition: calories 240, fat 12, fiber 3, carbs 5, protein 12

Avocado Salsa

You will make this over and over again! That's how tasty it is!

Preparation time: 10 minutes **Cooking time:** 0 minutes **Servings:** 4

Ingredients:

1 small red onion, chopped

2 avocados, pitted, peeled and chopped

3 jalapeno pepper, chopped

Salt and black pepper to the taste

2 tablespoons cumin powder

2 tablespoons lime juice

½ tomato, chopped

Directions:

1. In a bowl, mix onion with avocados, peppers, salt, black pepper, cumin, lime juice and tomato pieces and stir well.

2. Transfer this to a bowl and serve with toasted baguette slices as a keto appetizer.

Enjoy!

Nutrition: calories 120, fat 2, fiber 2, carbs 0.4, protein 4

Tasty Egg Chips

Do you want to impress everyone? Then, try these chips!

Preparation time: 5 minutes **Cooking time:** 10 minutes **Servings:** 2

Ingredients:½ tablespoon water

2 tablespoons parmesan, shredded

4 eggs whites

Salt and black pepper to the taste

Directions:

1. In a bowl, mix egg whites with salt, pepper and water and whisk well.

2. Spoon this into a muffin pan, sprinkle cheese on top, introduce in the oven at 400 degrees F and bake for 15 minutes.

3. Transfer egg white chips to a platter and serve with a keto dip on the side.

Enjoy!

Nutrition: calories 120, fat 2, fiber 1, carbs 2, protein 7

Chili Lime Chips

These crackers will impress you with their amazing taste!

Preparation time: 10 minutes **Cooking time:** 20 minutes **Servings:** 4

Ingredients:

1 cup almond flour

Salt and black pepper to the taste

1 and ½ teaspoons lime zest

1 teaspoon lime juice

1 egg

Directions:

1. In a bowl, mix almond flour with lime zest, lime juice and salt and stir.

2. Add egg and whisk well again.

3. Divide this into 4 parts, roll each into a ball and then spread well using a rolling pin.

4. Cut each into 6 triangles, place them all on a lined baking sheet, introduce in the oven at 350 degrees F and bake for 20 minutes.

Enjoy!

Nutrition: calories 90, fat 1, fiber 1, carbs 0.6, protein 3

Artichoke Dip

It's so rich and flavored!

Preparation time: 10 minutes **Cooking time:** 15 minutes **Servings:** 16

Ingredients:¼ cup sour cream

¼ cup heavy cream

¼ cup mayonnaise

¼ cup shallot, chopped

1 tablespoon olive oil

2 garlic cloves, minced

4 ounces cream cheese

½ cup parmesan cheese, grated

1 cup mozzarella cheese, shredded

4 ounces feta cheese, crumbled

1 tablespoon balsamic vinegar

28 ounces canned artichoke hearts, chopped

Salt and black pepper to the taste

10 ounces spinach, chopped

Directions:

1. Heat up a pan with the oil over medium heat, add shallot and garlic, stir and cook for 3 minutes.

2. Add heavy cream and cream cheese and stir.

3. Also add sour cream, parmesan, mayo, feta cheese and mozzarella cheese, stir and reduce heat.

4. Add artichoke, spinach, salt, pepper and vinegar, stir well, take off heat and transfer to a bowl.

5. Serve as a tasty keto dip.

Enjoy!

Nutrition: calories 144, fat 12, fiber 2, carbs 5, protein 5

FISH AND SEAFOOD

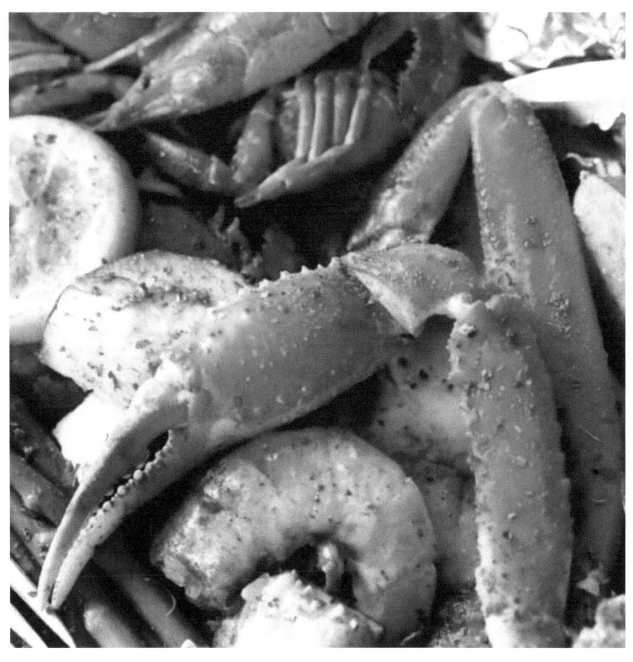

Crusted Salmon

The crust is wonderful!

Preparation time: 10 minutes **Cooking time:** 15 minutes **Servings:** 4

Ingredients:

3 garlic cloves, minced

2 pounds salmon fillet

Salt and black pepper to the taste

½ cup parmesan, grated

¼ cup parsley, chopped

Directions:

1. Place salmon on a lined baking sheet, season with salt and pepper, cover with a parchment paper, introduce in the oven at 425 degrees F and bake for 10 minutes.

2. Take fish out of the oven, sprinkle parmesan, parsley and garlic over fish, introduce in the oven again and cook for 5 minutes more.

3. Divide between plates and serve.

Enjoy!

Nutrition: calories 240, fat 12, fiber 1, carbs 0.6, protein 25

Sour Cream Salmon

It's perfect keto dish for a weekend meal!

Preparation time: 10 minutes **Cooking time:** 15 minutes **Servings:** 4

Ingredients:

4 salmon fillets

A drizzle of olive oil

Salt and black pepper to the taste

1/3 cup parmesan, grated

1 and ½ teaspoon mustard

½ cup sour cream

Directions:

1. Place salmon on a lined baking sheet, season with salt and pepper and drizzle the oil.

2. In a bowl, mix sour cream with parmesan, mustard, salt and pepper and stir well.

3. Spoon this sour cream mix over salmon, introduce in the oven at 350 degrees F and bake for 15 minutes.

4. Divide between plates and serve.

Enjoy!

Nutrition: calories 200, fat 6, fiber 1, carbs 4, protein 20

Grilled Salmon

This grilled salmon must be served with an avocado salsa!

Preparation time: 30 minutes **Cooking time:** 10 minutes **Servings:** 4

Ingredients:

4 salmon fillets

1 tablespoon olive oil

Salt and black pepper to the taste

1 teaspoon cumin, ground

1 teaspoon sweet paprika

½ teaspoon ancho chili powder

1 teaspoon onion powder

For the salsa:

1 small red onion, chopped

1 avocado, pitted, peeled and chopped

2 tablespoons cilantro, chopped

Juice from 2 limes

Salt and black pepper to the taste

Directions:

1. In a bowl, mix salt, pepper, chili powder, onion powder, paprika and cumin.

2. Rub salmon with this mix, drizzle the oil and rub again and cook on preheated grill for 4 minutes on each side.

3. Meanwhile, in a bowl, mix avocado with red onion, salt, pepper, cilantro and lime juice and stir.

4. Divide salmon between plates and top each fillet with avocado salsa.

Enjoy!

Nutrition: calories 300, fat 14, fiber 4, carbs 5, protein 20

Tasty Tuna Cakes

You just have to make these keto cakes for your family tonight!

Preparation time: 10 minutes **Cooking time:** 10 minutes **Servings:** 12

Ingredients:

15 ounces canned tuna, drain well and flaked

3 eggs

½ teaspoon dill, dried

1 teaspoon parsley, dried

½ cup red onion, chopped

1 teaspoon garlic powder

Salt and black pepper to the taste

Oil for frying

Directions:

1. In a bowl, mix tuna with salt, pepper, dill, parsley, onion, garlic powder and eggs and stir well.

2. Shape your cakes and place on a plate.

3. Heat up a pan with some oil over medium high heat, add tuna cakes, cook for 5 minutes on each side.

4. Divide between plates and serve.

Enjoy!

Nutrition: calories 140, fat 2, fiber 1, carbs 0.6, protein 6

Very Tasty Cod

Today, we recommend you to try a keto cod dish!

Preparation time: 10 minutes **Cooking time:** 20 minutes **Servings:** 4

Ingredients:

1 pound cod, cut into medium pieces

Salt and black pepper to the taste

2 green onions, chopped

3 garlic cloves, minced

3 tablespoons soy sauce

1 cup fish stock

1 tablespoons balsamic vinegar

1 tablespoon ginger, grated

½ teaspoon chili pepper, crushed

Directions:

1. Heat up a pan over medium high heat, add fish pieces and brown it a few minutes on each side.

2. Add garlic, green onions, salt, pepper, soy sauce, fish stock, vinegar, chili pepper and ginger, stir, cover, reduce heat and cook for 20 minutes.

3. Divide between plates and serve.

Enjoy!

Nutrition: calories 154, fat 3, fiber 0.5, carbs 4, protein 24

Tasty Sea Bass With Capers

It's a very tasty and easy dish to make at home when you are on a keto diet!

Preparation time: 10 minutes **Cooking time:** 15 minutes **Servings:** 4

Ingredients:

1 lemon, sliced

1 pound sea bass fillet

2 tablespoons capers

2 tablespoons dill

Salt and black pepper to the taste

Directions:

1. Put sea bass fillet into a baking dish, season with salt and pepper, add capers, dill and lemon slices on top.

2. Introduce in the oven at 350 degrees F and bake for 15 minutes.

3. Divide between plates and serve.

Enjoy!

Nutrition: calories 150, fat 3, fiber 2, carbs 0.7, protein 5

Cod With Arugula

It's an excellent keto meal that will be ready to serve in no time!

Preparation time: 10 minutes **Cooking time:** 20 minutes **Servings:** 2

Ingredients:

2 cod fillets

1 tablespoon olive oil

Salt and black pepper to the taste

Juice of 1 lemon

3 cup arugula

½ cup black olives, pitted and sliced

2 tablespoons capers

1 garlic clove, chopped

Directions:

1. Arrange fish fillets in a heatproof dish, season with salt, pepper, drizzle the oil and lemon juice, toss to coat, introduce in the oven at 450 degrees F and bake for 20 minutes.

2. In your food processor, mix arugula with salt, pepper, capers, olives and garlic and blend a bit.

3. Arrange fish on plates, top with arugula tapenade and serve. Enjoy!

Nutrition: calories 240, fat 5, fiber 3, carbs 3, protein 10

Baked Halibut And Veggies

You are going to love this great keto idea!

Preparation time: 10 minutes **Cooking time:** 35 minutes **Servings:** 2

Ingredients:

1 red bell pepper, roughly chopped

1 yellow bell pepper, roughly chopped

1 teaspoon balsamic vinegar

1 tablespoon olive oil

2 halibut fillets

2 cups baby spinach

Salt and black pepper to the taste

1 teaspoon cumin

Directions:

1. In a bowl, mix bell peppers with salt, pepper, half of the oil and the vinegar, toss to coat well and transfer to a baking dish.

2. Introduce in the oven at 400 degrees F and bake for 20 minutes.

3. Heat up a pan with the rest of the oil over medium heat, add fish, season with salt, pepper and cumin and brown on all sides.

4. Take the baking dish out of the oven, add spinach, stir gently and divide the whole mix between plates.

5. Add fish on the side, sprinkle some more salt and pepper and serve.

Enjoy!

Nutrition: calories 230, fat 12, fiber 1, carbs 4, protein 9

Tasty Fish Curry

Have you ever tried a Ketogenic curry? Then you should really pay attention next!

Preparation time: 10 minutes **Cooking time:** 25 minutes **Servings:** 4

Ingredients:

4 white fish fillets

½ teaspoon mustard seeds

Salt and black pepper to the taste

2 green chilies, chopped

1 teaspoon ginger, grated

1 teaspoon curry powder

¼ teaspoon cumin, ground

4 tablespoons coconut oil

1 small red onion, chopped

1 inch turmeric root, grated

¼ cup cilantro

1 and ½ cups coconut cream

3 garlic cloves, minced

Directions:

1. Heat up a pot with half of the coconut oil over medium heat, add mustard seeds and cook for 2 minutes.

2. Add ginger, onion and garlic, stir and cook for 5 minutes.

3. Add turmeric, curry powder, chilies and cumin, stir and cook for 5 minutes more.

4. Add coconut milk, salt and pepper, stir, bring to a boil and cook for 15 minutes.

5. Heat up another pan with the rest of the oil over medium heat, add fish, stir and cook for 3 minutes.

6. Add this to the curry sauce, stir and cook for 5 minutes more.

7. Add cilantro, stir, divide into bowls and serve.

Enjoy!

Nutrition: calories 500, fat 34, fiber 7, carbs 6, protein 44

Delicious Shrimp

It's an easy and tasty idea for dinner!

Preparation time: 10 minutes **Cooking time:** 10 minutes **Servings:** 4

Ingredients:

2 tablespoons olive oil

1 tablespoon ghee

1 pound shrimp, peeled and deveined

2 tablespoons lemon juice

2 tablespoons garlic, minced

1 tablespoon lemon zest

Salt and black pepper to the taste

Directions:

1. Heat up a pan with the oil and the ghee over medium high heat, add shrimp and cook for 2 minutes.

2. Add garlic, stir and cook for 4 minutes more.

3. Add lemon juice, lemon zest, salt and pepper, stir, take off heat and serve.

Enjoy!

Nutrition: calories 149, fat 1, fiber 3, carbs 1, protein 6

DESSERT

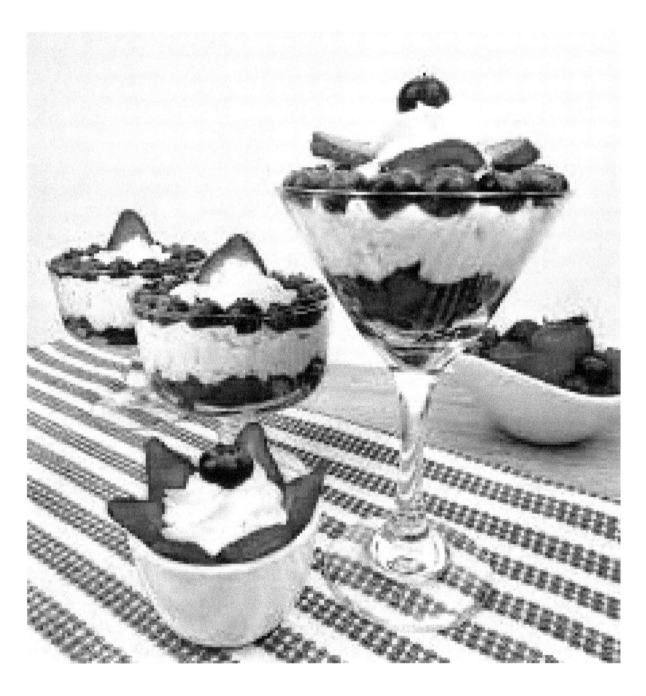

Simple Peanut Butter Fudge

You only need a few ingredients to make this tasty keto dessert!

Preparation time: 2 hours and 10 minutes **Cooking time:** 2 minutes

Servings: 12

Ingredients:

1 cup peanut butter, unsweetened

¼ cup almond milk

2 teaspoons vanilla stevia

1 cup coconut oil

A pinch of salt

For the topping:

2 tablespoons swerve

2 tablespoons melted coconut oil

¼ cup cocoa powder

Directions:

1. In a heat proof bowl, mix peanut butter with 1 cup coconut oil, stir and heat up in your microwave until it melts.

2. Add a pinch of salt, almond milk and stevia, stir well everything and pour into a lined loaf pan.

3. Keep in the fridge for 2 hours and then slice it.

4. In a bowl, mix 2 tablespoons melted coconut with cocoa powder and swerve and stir very well.

5. Drizzle the sauce over your peanut butter fudge and serve. Enjoy!

Nutrition: calories 265, fat 23, fiber 2, carbs 4, protein 6

Lemon Mousse

This is so refreshing and delicious!

Preparation time: 10 minutes **Cooking time:** 0 minutes **Servings:** 5

Ingredients:

1 cup heavy cream

A pinch of salt

1 teaspoon lemon stevia

¼ cup lemon juice

8 ounces mascarpone cheese

Directions:

1. In a bowl, mix heavy cream with mascarpone and lemon juice and stir using your mixer.

2. Add a pinch of salt and stevia and blend everything.

3. Divide into dessert glasses and keep in the fridge until you serve.

Enjoy!

Nutrition: calories 265, fat 27, fiber 0, carbs 2, protein 4

Vanilla Ice Cream

Try this keto ice cream on a summer day!

Preparation time: 3 hours and 10 minutes **Cooking time:** 0 minutes

Servings:

6

Ingredients:

4 eggs, yolks and whites separated

¼ teaspoon cream of tartar

½ cup swerve

1 tablespoon vanilla extract

1 and ¼ cup heavy whipping cream

Directions:

1. In a bowl, mix egg whites with cream of tartar and swerve and stir using your mixer.

2. In another bowl, whisk cream with vanilla extract and blend very well.

3. Combine the 2 mixtures and stir gently.

4. In another bowl, whisk egg yolks very well and then add the two egg whites mix.

5. Stir gently, pour this into a container and keep in the freezer for 3 hours before serving your ice cream.

Enjoy!

Nutrition: calories 243, fat 22, fiber 0, carbs 2, protein 4

Cheesecake Squares

They look so good!

Preparation time: 10 minutes **Cooking time:** 20 minutes **Servings:** 9

Ingredients:

5 ounces coconut oil, melted

½ teaspoon baking powder

4 tablespoons swerve

1 teaspoon vanilla

4 ounces cream cheese

6 eggs

½ cup blueberries

Directions:

1. In a bowl, mix coconut oil with eggs, cream cheese, vanilla, swerve and baking powder and blend using an immersion blender.

2. Fold blueberries, pour everything into a square baking dish, introduce in the oven at 320 degrees F and bake for 20 minutes.

3. Leave you cake to cool down, slice into squares and serve. Enjoy!

Nutrition: calories 220, fat 2, fiber 0.5, carbs 2, protein 4

Tasty Brownies

These flourless keto brownies are excellent!

Preparation time: 10 minutes **Cooking time:** 20 minutes **Servings:** 12

Ingredients:

6 ounces coconut oil, melted

6 eggs

3 ounces cocoa powder

2 teaspoons vanilla

½ teaspoon baking powder

4 ounces cream cheese

5 tablespoons swerve

Directions:

1. In a blender, mix eggs with coconut oil, cocoa powder, baking powder, vanilla, cream cheese and swerve and stir using a mixer.

2. Pour this into a lined baking dish, introduce in the oven at 350 degrees F and bake for 20 minutes.

3. Slice into rectangle pieces when their cold and serve.

Enjoy!

Nutrition: calories 178, fat 14, fiber 2, carbs 3, protein 5

Chocolate Pudding

This pudding is so tasty!

Preparation time: 50 minutes **Cooking time:** 5 minutes **Servings:** 2

Ingredients:

2 tablespoons water

1 tablespoon gelatin

2 tablespoons maple syrup

½ teaspoon stevia powder

2 tablespoons cocoa powder

1 cup coconut milk

Directions:

1. Heat up a pan with the coconut milk over medium heat, add stevia and cocoa powder and stir well.

2. In a bowl, mix gelatin with water, stir well and add to the pan.

3. Stir well, add maple syrup, whisk again, divide into ramekins and keep in the fridge for 45 minutes.

4. Serve cold.

Enjoy!

Nutrition: calories 140, fat 2, fiber 2, carbs 4, protein 4

Vanilla Parfaits

These will make you fell amazing!

Preparation time: 10 minutes **Cooking time:** 0 minutes **Servings:** 4

Ingredients:

14 ounces canned coconut milk

1 teaspoon vanilla extract

10 drops stevia

4 ounces berries

2 tablespoons walnuts, chopped

Directions:

1. In a bowl, mix coconut milk with stevia and vanilla extract and whisk using your mixer.

2. IN another bowl, mix berries with walnuts and stir.

3. Spoon half of vanilla coconut mix into 4 jars, add a layer of berries and top with the rest of the vanilla mix.

4. Top with berries and walnuts mix, introduce in the fridge until you serve it.

Enjoy!

Nutrition: calories 400, fat 23, fiber 4, carbs 6, protein 7

Simple Avocado Pudding

This is so easy to make at home and it follows keto principles!

Preparation time: 10 minutes **Cooking time:** 0 minutes **Servings:** 4

Ingredients:

2 avocados, pitted, peeled and chopped

2 teaspoons vanilla extract

80 drops stevia

1 tablespoon lime juice

14 ounces canned coconut milk

Directions:

1. In your blender, mix avocado with coconut milk, vanilla extract, stevia and lime juice, blend well, spoon into dessert bowls and keep in the fridge until you serve it.

Enjoy!

Nutrition: calories 150, fat 3, fiber 3, carbs 5, protein 6

Mint Delight

It has such a fresh texture and taste!

Preparation time: 2 hours and 10 minutes **Cooking time:** 0 minutes

Servings:

3

Ingredients:½ cup coconut oil, melted

3 stevia drops

1 tablespoon cocoa powder

For the pudding:

1 teaspoon peppermint oil

14 ounces canned coconut milk

1 avocado, pitted, peeled and chopped

10 drops stevia

Directions:

1. In a bowl, mix coconut oil with cocoa powder and 3 drops stevia, stir well, transfer to a lined container and keep in the fridge for 1 hour.

2. Chop this into small pieces and leave aside for now.

3. In your blender, mix coconut milk with avocado, 10 drops stevia and peppermint oil and pulse well.

4. Add chocolate chips, fold them gently, divide pudding into bowls and keep in the fridge for 1 more hour.

Enjoy!

Nutrition: calories 140, fat 3, fiber 2, carbs 3, protein 4

Amazing Coconut Pudding

You've got to love this keto pudding!

Preparation time: 10 minutes **Cooking time:** 10 minutes **Servings:** 4

Ingredients:

1 and 2/3 cups coconut milk

1 tablespoon gelatin

6 tablespoons swerve

3 egg yolks

½ teaspoon vanilla extract

Directions:

1. In a bowl, mix gelatin with 1 tablespoon coconut milk, stir well and leave aside for now.

2. Put the rest of the milk into a pan and heat up over medium heat.

3. Add swerve, stir and cook for 5 minutes.

4. In a bowl, mix egg yolks with the hot coconut milk and vanilla extract, stir well and return everything to the pan.

5. Cook for 4 minutes, add gelatin and stir well.

6. Divide this into 4 ramekins and keep your pudding in the fridge until you serve it.

Enjoy!

Nutrition: calories 140, fat 2, fiber 0, carbs 2, protein 2

CPSIA information can be obtained
at www.ICGtesting.com
Printed in the USA
BVHW052137030521
606339BV00014B/2413